Health Care Careers

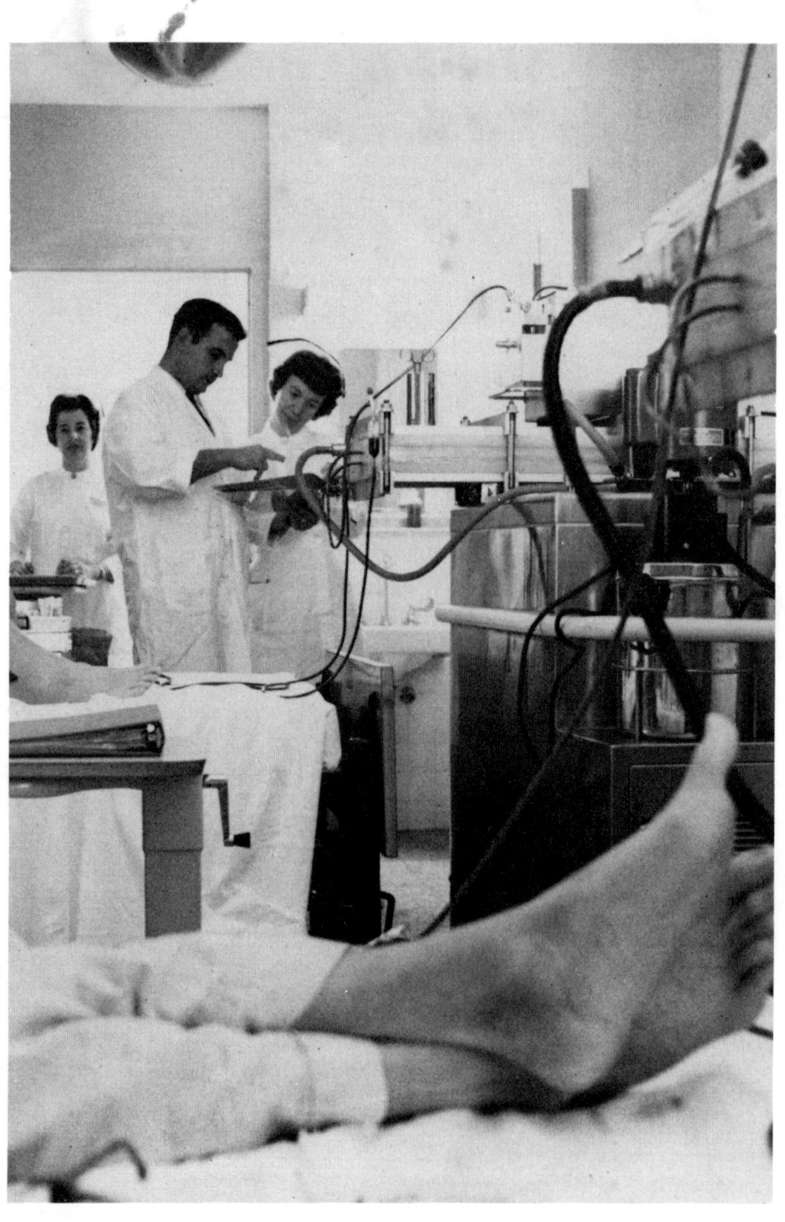

Today's complex hospitals require the services of doctors, nurses, aides, technicians who understand complicated equipment, and many, many others.

Health Care Careers

by Eleanor Kay, R.N.

illustrated with photographs

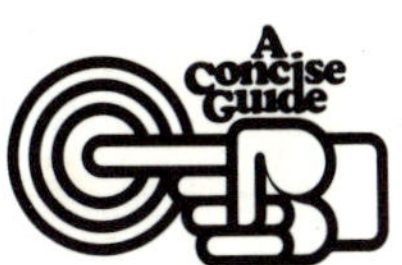

FRANKLIN WATTS, INC. • NEW YORK

1973

Cover design by One + One Studio

Photographs courtesy of:
Armed Forces Institute of Pathology, pp. 24; Brooklyn Longshoremen's Medical Center, pp. 17; Duke University, Durham, N.C., title, pps. 14, 20, 35, 45, 61; Montefiore Hospital, Pittsburgh, Pa., pps. 11, 48, 51; National Institutes of Health, pps. 5, 41, 56; North Carolina Baptist Hospital, pp. 29; Samaritan Health Service, pp. 8.

Library of Congress Cataloging in Publication Data

Kay, Eleanor.
Health care careers.

(A Concise guide)
1. Medical personnel–United States–Education.
I. Title. [DNLM: 1. Allied health personnel.
2. Health occupations. W 21 K23h 1973]
R745.K38 362.1'023 72-8881
ISBN 0-531-02607-8

Printed in the United States of America
2 3 4 5

Contents

Introduction

What do you think of when you hear the words "health care"? A doctor in white? A nurse walking softly into a hospital room on rubber-soled shoes?

These people are a vital part of health care, of course. But you might be amazed to learn of the many others who are needed to return people to good health as quickly as possible. If you were to spend about a week as a hospital patient, chances are at the end of that time you would have seen or heard about the following people: a doctor, a professional nurse, a practical nurse, a radiology technician, a medical technologist, a nursing aide, a pharmacist, a housekeeper, a dietician, an operating room technician, an inhalation therapist, a speech pathologist, a hospital administrator, a physician's associate, a social worker, a medical record librarian, and more.

If you have considered a career in the health care field, you have probably thought first of becoming a doctor or nurse. Both of these careers require long training. But the health care field offers many other opportunities besides nursing or medicine. If you are interested, *now* is the time to prepare yourself.

This book will introduce you to a number of possible careers in health care, explaining the types of work involved and what education and training are needed. With few exceptions, these careers require at least a high school education or its equivalent. Many require a college degree.

For many careers in the health care field, federal or state funds are available for both the educational programs and living expenses. If you are interested in a particular area, you should seek information about financial assistance from the school you wish to apply to or from the national association that covers your particular field of interest. At the end of each chapter are found the names and addresses of the related national associations, as well as general admission requirements for the programs and typical courses of study. The listed courses of study are not intended to be complete but only to give the interested student an idea of the subjects to be studied. The name of the institution from which the partial curriculum was taken is also listed.

Perhaps there is a place for you in this important and growing field, which for a long time has needed more and more qualified, interested people. A career in health care can be exciting, challenging, and rewarding.

Professional Nursing

Edith McGuirk is a head nurse in a hospital. As head nurse she is responsible for planning a program of care for each patient on her unit. Working with the doctors, she keeps a careful check on each patient's progress, and she tries to anticipate his or her needs. If the patient is to have a complete X-ray study, she explains the procedure to him. If he needs surgery, she, along with the doctors and others, tells the patient what is to be done and what the expected physical reaction will be.

Throughout a routine day Edith McGuirk will meet many different situations that she must cope with quickly and efficiently. Her skill may make a great deal of difference in a patient's battle for good health. It is not an easy job, but her educational background in nursing and her experience have given her the ability to do it with confidence.

Edith is one of thousands of registered professional nurses, male and female, in the United States. She graduated from the University of Michigan, with a four-year nursing baccalaureate degree, and gained additional experience at medical center hospitals in California, Oregon, and North Carolina.

Professional nursing today is far different from what it was years ago. Today's nurse is constantly involved in an expanding role. The modern practice of nursing requires more and more educational preparation so that the nurse may understand and contribute to new methods of care and treatment.

Today's professional nurses practice in many different areas. A nurse may work in a rural community as a family nurse practitioner, giving complete health care to the entire family, and assuming a great many duties usually taken care of by the physician. She may be a pediatric nurse, caring for newborn infants and their mothers. She may work in drug programs, community centers, mobile clinics, diagnostic centers for preventive health care needs, in industry, on board ships, and in many other non-hospital areas.

Within the hospital, the nurse may work on the wards, in the emergency room, the operating room, the cardiac care unit, and the nursing office. Some nurses have taken postgraduate programs and become nurse anesthetists. Others take additional education courses and become nurse-teachers.

One fast-growing specialty for the professional nurse is nurse-midwife. The nurse-midwife is a registered nurse who, through a program of study and clinical experience, has learned to care for mothers and babies throughout the maternity cycle. She supervises the care for the mother during pregnancy and is with her during labor. She manages the whole process of labor and delivery and helps the mother to care for herself and the newborn child. The nurse-midwife works with an obstetrician who is available to her for consultation.

There are three basic programs for a nursing education in the United States. Each one trains the young man or woman to become licensed as a professional nurse. But there are differences in the programs and in the futures they can provide. A student interested in becoming a nurse should choose carefully the program best suited to his or her interests, abilities, and goals. It is often a difficult choice.

The American Nursing Association favors the four-year college or university affiliated baccalaureate program for men and women seeking a career in professional nursing. Throughout this program the student will learn much about interpersonal relationships that will be important in a nursing career. In addition, the education in the sciences prepares the student to understand more completely basic principles of science and its relationship to the patient's total needs. Many of the courses during the prenursing program are taken with other health care team members, such as medical, dental, and pharmacy students, so that a relationship is established early among students who

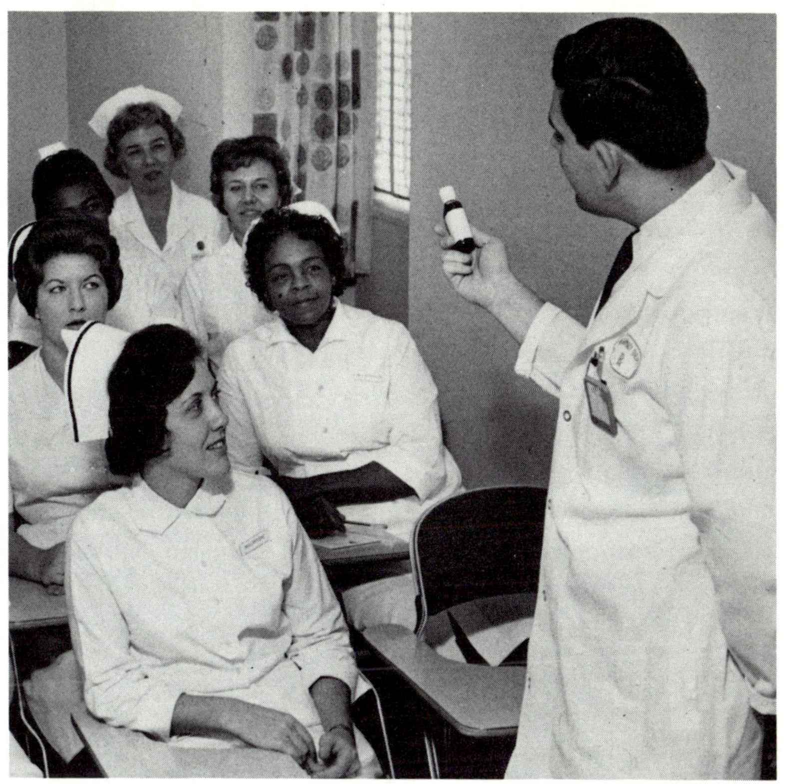

The modern practice of nursing requires preparation in many areas.

will one day work together as licensed professionals. The nursing student receives a college baccalaureate degree upon graduation from this program.

The three-year diploma program, offered primarily through hospitals, also provides an excellent opportunity for a young man or woman to develop professionally. However, it offers no college degree upon completion.

The associated degree program, offered by community colleges, prepares the graduate to practice basic nursing. This two-year course is basic nursing and encourages the student to go on with his or her education in order to obtain a baccalaureate degree in nursing at a later date.

Upon completion of any nursing program, the graduate is required to pass a licensing exam in order to become a registered professional nurse.

The costs of these three programs vary. The cost of the four-year program is that of a college education. Community colleges are often tuition-free. Fees vary widely in the diploma program, according to the hospital where the program is taken.

A student interested in a nursing career should, with the help of a high school advisor, examine the programs carefully to find the one best suited to his or her abilities.

REQUIREMENTS: high school education

COURSE OF STUDY

Baccalaureate program: English, Mathematical Sciences, Physical Education, Languages, Social Sciences, Humanities and Fine Arts, Natural Sciences, Physiology, Bacteriology, Microbiology, Dynamics of Human Development, Pathological Processes, Concepts of Community Health, Leadership, and various nursing courses (University of North Carolina at Chapel Hill School of Nursing)

Diploma program: Chemistry, Microbiology, English, Anatomy/Physiology, General Psychology, Pharmacology, Nutrition, Sociology, Ethics, Marriage Guidance, and various nursing courses (Mercy Hospital School of Nursing, Scranton, Pennsylvania)

Associated degree program: English, Physical Education, Psychology, Anatomy and Physiology, Art or Music Survey, Speech Fundamentals, Bacteriology, Sociology, General Organic and Biological Chemistry, and various nursing courses (Bronx Community College, New York)

NATIONAL ASSOCIATION:

National League for Nursing, Inc.
10 Columbus Circle
New York, New York 10019

Practical Nursing

Hilda Evans reported for duty and waited for her assignment from the head nurse. She had completed her practical nursing course and obtained her license by examination some months before. By now she had lost count of the number of beds she had made, the baths she had given, and the assistance she had provided to patients who needed help in walking, getting out of bed, completing blood examinations, and coming and going to and from X-ray and other areas. She had already assisted on two emergencies — Code 5 cardiac arrests. Both patients' hearts had stopped working, and they had required immediate emergency care. Calls had been placed to the emergency team, and the response in both situations had been within seconds. Hilda had worked the "cart" — a portable table that holds all the drugs, syringes, and emergency equipment necessary for the doctors and nurses to use on the patient. She had kept careful records of the medications used, taking them from the various compartments and quickly giving them to the assisting nurse during the tense moments.

During World War II, the great need for many more people to help care for the thousands of patients in hospitals all over the country prompted the development of a rapid program for nursing assistants. Regular hospital nurses were short-handed because thousands of them were in the armed forces.

The first training programs for practical nurses were very basic and short. Young women mainly took courses at hospitals, vocational schools, and the local chapters of the Red Cross. With little training, the assistance they were able to give patients was satisfactory for that time. However, as more complex methods of treatment were developed, a more rigorous program was needed for educating people in this fast-growing field.

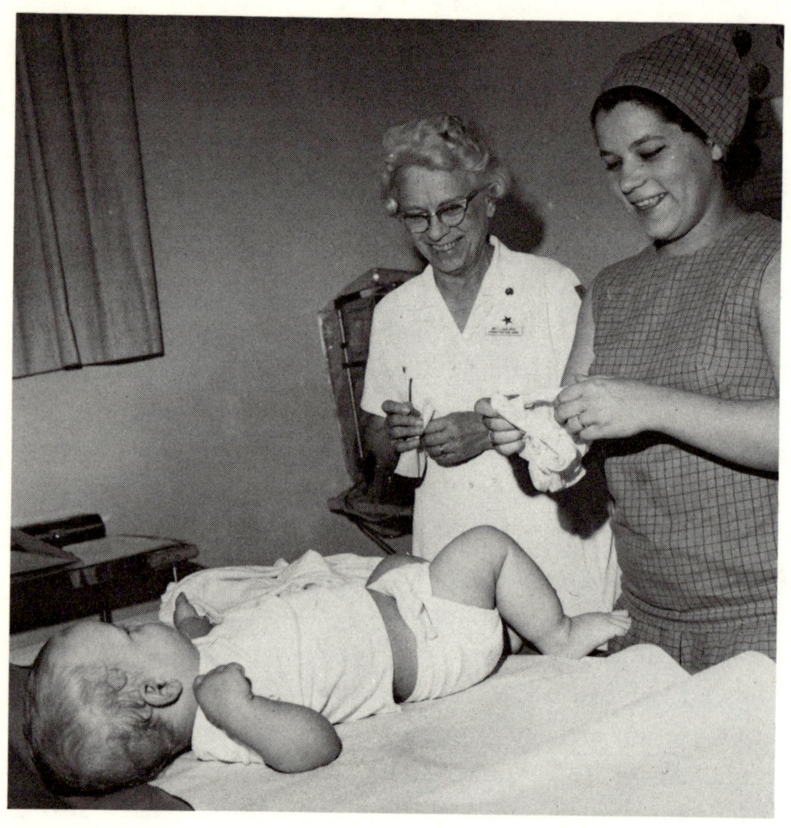

The practical nurse (in white uniform) at work

Today, practical nursing programs are usually one year long. However, in some states the programs may be longer. They are given at technical institutions or hospitals. Although the costs vary, they are considerably lower than any of the programs for professional nurses.

During training the practical nursing student is assigned to units within a specific hospital. Under professional nursing supervision, he or she gives the patients the care that has been taught in classroom lectures and demonstrations.

On completion of the program, practical nurses are required to take an examination in the particular state in which they are trained. If they pass the test, they receive licenses to practice. The test examines the student not only on the materials learned in classroom teaching, but also on the practical application of that knowledge. It is designed to make the applicant demonstrate his or her understanding of the various skills taught and worked with during the training period.

After graduation and the examination, the female practical nurse wears a white uniform with the practical nurse insignia on the sleeve. Male practical nurses wear white uniforms similar to those of hospital interns, also with the insignia.

Practical nurses work in hospitals, clinics, nursing homes, community centers, and other areas related to health care. They assume some responsibility for patient care, but are always supervised by professional nurses.

REQUIREMENTS: high school education

COURSE OF STUDY: Nutritional Practices, Community Health, Body Structure and Organ Functions, Types and Symptoms of Disease and Illness, Medicines and their administration, Hygienic Procedures of Patient Care (Durham Technical Institute, Durham, North Carolina)

NATIONAL ASSOCIATION:

National League for Nursing, Inc.
10 Columbus Circle
New York, New York 10019

Medical Technologist

Sandy Rosen looked through the microscope at the blood sample. The number on the edge of the slide was the same as the number on the laboratory sheet on his work table. He had placed both numbers there himself this morning after he had drawn blood from a patient's arm.

Across the workbench from Sandy sat Barbara Powers, recently employed at the laboratory to do special studies on blood.

After a time Sandy looked up from his work. "Barbara, I've got a number of immature cells here with a high concentration of hemoglobin," he said. "I'll give you a sample to analyze."

Sandy took a clean test tube and transferred some of the blood sample carefully into it by using a small glass pipette and tube.

When completely examined, Sandy's blood sample showed that the patient had an infection; his body was not only producing a high count of white blood cells to fight the infection, but the infection was depleting his red cells in the process. In addition, the test for hemoglobin — a study to show iron content — was considerably lower than it should be.

Barbara's examination of the blood showed that many of the patient's red cells were immature but contained a great deal of hemoglobin. The results of both tests together produced a picture of a patient suffering from an infection manufacturing red cells that were entering his circulatory system before they were mature enough to carry out their responsibilities. They carried more hemoglobin content than fully developed cells would normally have.

These results were given to the doctor who was chief of the laboratory staff at the hospital. He would discuss the possibilities of diagnosis and treatment with the patient's own doctor.

Barbara and Sandy are medical technologists. In hospital

be replaced twice a week with a fresh sterilized set. Pete made a notation on his treatment sheet of the time, the amount of medication he had placed in the machine, and how well the patient had responded, so that other technicians would have the data to review before they started the next treatment.

Inhalation therapy dates only from the late 1950's. It replaced an original treatment carried out by physicians and nurses called "postural drainage." However, since this method required a patient to hang his head down for a time, it was often very difficult for an ill patient to do.

As new techniques and machines were developed, the need for postural drainage disappeared and the respirator machines took over the job more effectively. The first inhalation technicians were taught "on-the-job" by nurses and doctors. Then the techniques and machinery became more and more complex, offering new methods to help breathing problems of even the tiniest premature baby. The advancement in technology required technicians to be more prepared than any on-the-job program could provide. Inhalation therapy schools, under the auspices of the American Medical Association, began to develop, and soon a detailed curriculum was designed.

In most major teaching institutions, inhalation therapy programs are under the direction of the Department of Anesthesiology and are about two years long. On completion the therapist must take an examination and become licensed as an Inhalation Therapy Technician before he can practice.

REQUIREMENTS: high school education

COURSE OF STUDY: Biology, Chemistry, Grammar, Mathematics, Blueprint Reading and Sketching, Nursing Arts, Anatomy and Physiology, Pharmacology, Oral Communications, Technical Writing, Electricity, Microbiology and Pathology, Applied Psychology, Social Sciences (Durham Technical Institute, Durham, North Carolina)

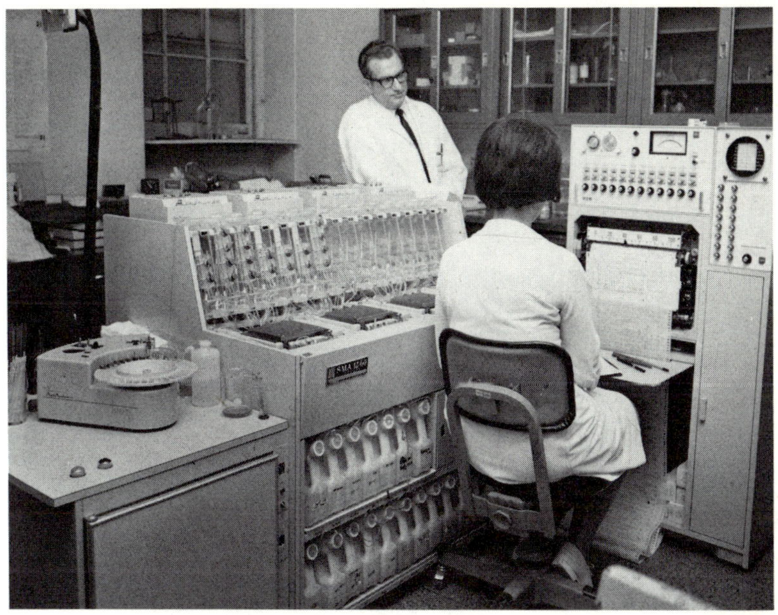

In the hospital laboratory

laboratories, they perform chemical, microscopic, and bacteriological examinations, as well as other tests.

Most hospitals maintain separate laboratories to carry out tests in various areas. The blood bank is primarily concerned with the examination and study of blood typing for transfusions. The cytology laboratory is principally used for the testing of cells shed by body tissue. For instance, the Papanicolaou test examines specimens for cancer cells. In the histology laboratory technologists examine sections of tissue removed by surgery or a similar procedure to determine cell structure and the arrangement of the cells in the specimen. The hematology laboratory, where Sandy and Barbara work, is concerned with the search for abnormalities in the blood.

Medical technologists must have a minimum of three years of college study. In order to become a registered medical technologist, the student takes a twelve-month course in an American

Medical Association accredited school. Upon graduation from the technology school, the student takes an examination. If he passes, he is certified by the Registry of Medical Technologists, American Society of Clinical Pathologists (ASCP).

There are other categories of laboratory personnel now active within hospitals and laboratories throughout the country.

Cytotechnologists specialize in the screening of slides in search of abnormalities that indicate cancer. This work requires two years of college, and twelve months training at an American Medical Association approved school of cytotechnology, the last six months at the school or in a cytology laboratory.

Laboratory assistants who perform many of the simpler diagnostic tests and laboratory procedures are required to have a high school diploma and a one-year course in a hospital laboratory or laboratory school approved for training.

Histology technicians cut and stain the tissue to be examined by the pathologist. They must have a high school diploma and one year's experience in supervised training in a clinical pathology laboratory or junior college program.

Although there has been a great surge in the development of machines that can carry out a number of tests on a number of samples at one time, the demand for laboratory technicians grows each day.

REQUIREMENTS: high school education

COURSE OF STUDY: English, Mathematics, Modern Civilization, Language, Social Science, Physical Education, Chemistry, Zoology, Bacteriology, Microbiology, Hematology, Tissue, Biochemistry, Basal Metabolism, Ethics, and Laboratory Management (medical technologist, University of North Carolina)

NATIONAL ASSOCIATION:

Registry of Medical Technologists
of the American Society of Clinical Pathologists
Box 4872, Chicago, Illinois 60680

Radiology Technician

Mary Boder is a licensed radiology technician. Her prime responsibility is to take correctly the various X-ray studies that doctors order for their patients.

Taking an X-ray picture is not unlike taking a regular photograph, but it is far more complex. The X-ray machine will produce pictures only if the technician has carefully measured the thickness of the particular part being studied; made adjustments in setting the voltage used and in the time sequence; and properly positioned the patient for the required views.

In addition, the technician must understand the size film that is needed, the safety precautions for the patient, and many other related details. So, it is not quite as simple as focusing the camera and pushing a button.

In order to learn how to do all of this, a radiology technician must go to school. Most radiology courses are two years long, and most schools do not charge tuition, although the student must pay for books, uniforms, and room and board.

Some technicians enter radiation therapy, another branch of radiology, by taking additional courses in radiation therapy methods. Since this therapy is usually given to patients with tumors or other types of disorders, the technician learns about these diseases and their effects on body tissue, as well as the effects of radiation upon both diseased and healthy tissue.

Radiology programs are supervised by physician radiologists. These are doctors who have finished their medical training and have specialized in the field of radiology, or, as it is commonly known, X-ray. On completion of the program, the graduate must pass an examination to determine his comprehension and skill. Then he has earned the right to carry a license denoting him as a licensed radiology technician.

Radiology technicians are much in demand throughout the

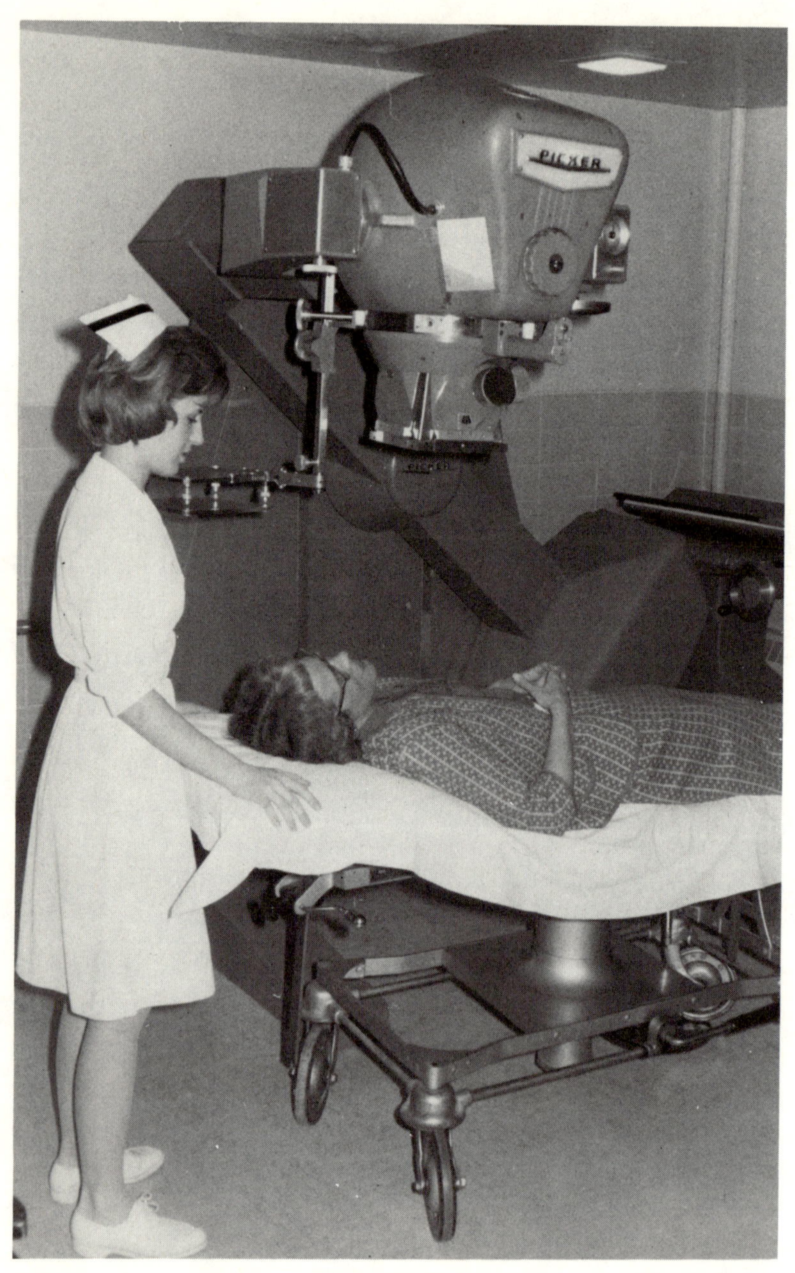

Radiology technicians are much in demand.

health care field. They are needed in community clinics, mobile radiology units, hospitals, doctors' offices, in the armed forces, and for many organizations providing radiological health services to millions of people the world over.

REQUIREMENTS: high school education

COURSE OF STUDY: Anatomy and Physiology, Darkroom Chemistry, Physics, Principles of Radiographic Exposure, Medical Terminology, Pediatric Radiology, Nursing Procedures Pertinent to Radiology, Radiographic Positioning, Protection of Patients and Personnel, Film Critique, Radiation Therapy, Equipment Maintenance (Georgetown University Hospital, Washington, D.C.)

NATIONAL ASSOCIATION:

The American Society of Radiologic Technologists
645 N. Michigan Avenue, Rm. 620
Chicago, Illinois 60611

Physician

Dr. Richard Ebling looked at the chart of the newest admission to the hospital unit. He read over some of the notations made by the patient's physician and other health care team members. Reading the progress notes, the X-ray reports, the laboratory slips, the history information sheet, the report of the physical examination carried out by the intern, plus the nursing notes kept on the patient since his admission, Dr. Ebling had a concise picture of the new patient — without yet having met him.

Following his own examination of the patient, Dr. Ebling confirmed the intern's findings. As the resident physician of this hospital floor, it is Dr. Ebling's responsibility to check and evaluate the work of the interns.

The doctor wrote a lengthy progress note on the patient's chart, detailing his physical examination findings and his diagnosis and subsequent treatment suggestions. He noted that the patient's attending physician had also written a lengthy note, and that much of it agreed with his own findings and suggestions.

Next, Dr. Ebling called the patient's doctor and discussed orders that both physicians thought best for care and treatment. Then Dr. Ebling wrote the orders into the chart so that the unit staff could carry them out. The doctor checked off the patient's name in his record book and saw that he still had fourteen other people to see on his rounds.

After completing premedical and medical educational programs, doctors work in hospitals as interns and then as residents to further their skills and knowledge. Students also work in a hospital during their last two years of medical school. This approach has been in practice for some years and has proven beneficial in the education of doctors.

Medical students are closely supervised by the intern, a

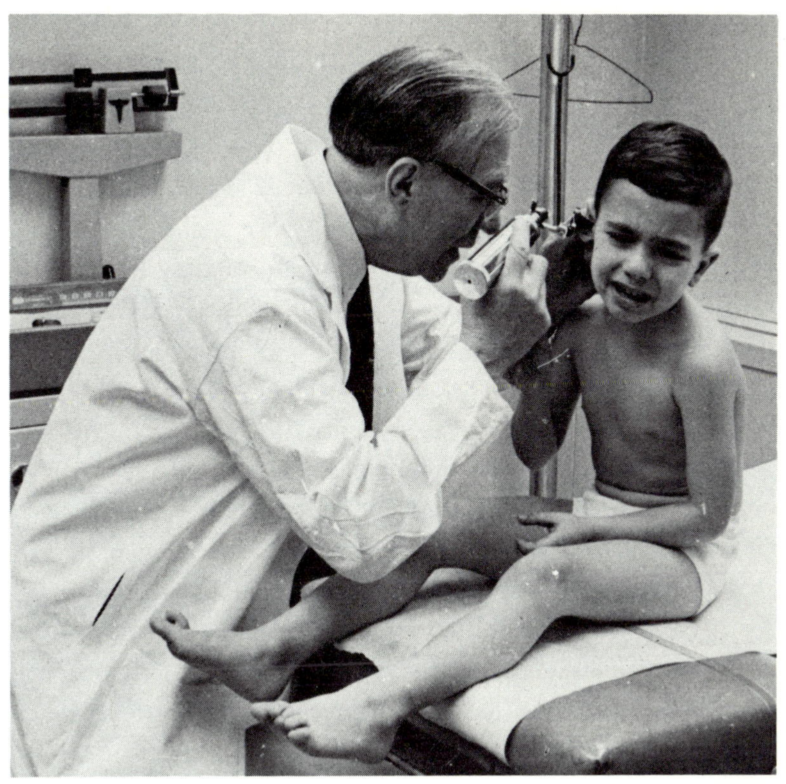

This doctor is examining a rather unwilling young patient.

graduate doctor, and the resident physician, who is a graduate doctor with greater experience. The residents and interns, in turn, are supervised by attending physicians. These are people who hold positions of responsibility in the overall medical management of the hospital, such as the chief of surgery or chief of medicine. Along with the chiefs, other attending physicians hold appointments to various services that they specialize in, and they also teach and supervise young doctors.

All teaching hospitals have programs of teaching, research, and patient care as their basic responsibilities. All staff doctors, regardless of their particular area of interest in medicine, participate in this program to aid in the education of the younger physicians.

Young men or women interested in becoming doctors should prepare themselves for an arduous time of study. Most medical schools require at least three years of premedical study in a college, with satisfactory grades and high standing in the class. Medical school itself is a four-year, rigorous period. On graduation, most students take a one- or two-year internship, followed by a two- or three-year (or longer) residency program. The total time of study for a physician is approximately eleven years.

During that time the young physician will have been exposed to all areas of medicine and will probably have fixed on an area of interest. Today, due to the increasing amount of data constantly being uncovered and the vast amount of knowledge already unearthed in health care, many young medical students are able to pick their area of specialization by their junior year of medical school, and thus can spend their time more profitably in that specific area.

REQUIREMENTS: at least three years premedical college study

COURSE OF STUDY: Basic sciences such as Gross Anatomy, Histology, Neuroscience, and Genetics. Clinical instruction in Medicine and Surgery, Obstetrics and Gynecology, Pediatrics and Psychiatry. Major programs offered in preclinical sciences, Medicine and Surgery, Obstetrics and Gynecology, Pediatrics, and the Neurological Sciences and Psychiatry (University of Vermont, College of Medicine)

NATIONAL ASSOCIATION:

Council on Medical Education
American Medical Association
535 N. Dearborn Street
Chicago, Illinois 60610

Inhalation Therapist

The intern who had first examined Dr. Ebling's patient had made a notation on his chart that the man's lungs had high squeaking sounds significant of congestion. A chest X-ray showed that the lungs were indeed congested. Dr. Ebling and the attending physician decided to have the patient begin inhalation therapy treatments to help clear the congestion before possible surgery. This would be helpful even if an operation was not scheduled.

Pete Weiss, Inhalation Therapist, was assigned to give the patient his first treatment. Pete had taken his training at the University of Michigan Inhalation Therapy School and had come to this hospital after working at the University of Michigan for two years after graduation.

The Inhalation Therapy Treatment slip for the patient read I.P.P.B. This is hospital jargon for "intermittent positive pressure breathing." The machine, using a small plastic mouthpiece, assists the patient in taking very deep breaths that force air deeply into the lung tissue. By doing so the circulation within the lung becomes more pronounced, thus breaking up the congestion of mucous and fluid. Once broken into particles, the congestion is absorbed into the circulatory system and excreted through the body or coughed up during treatment.

Pete wheeled the I.P.P.B. machine to the patient's room. He checked with the head nurse to make sure he could have fifteen uninterrupted minutes to carry out the treatment. He also made arrangements to have the treatment repeated twice more during the day.

When the treatment was over, Pete took the machine with him, but left behind in a plastic bag the connecting tubing and small mouthpiece that the patient had used. These items would

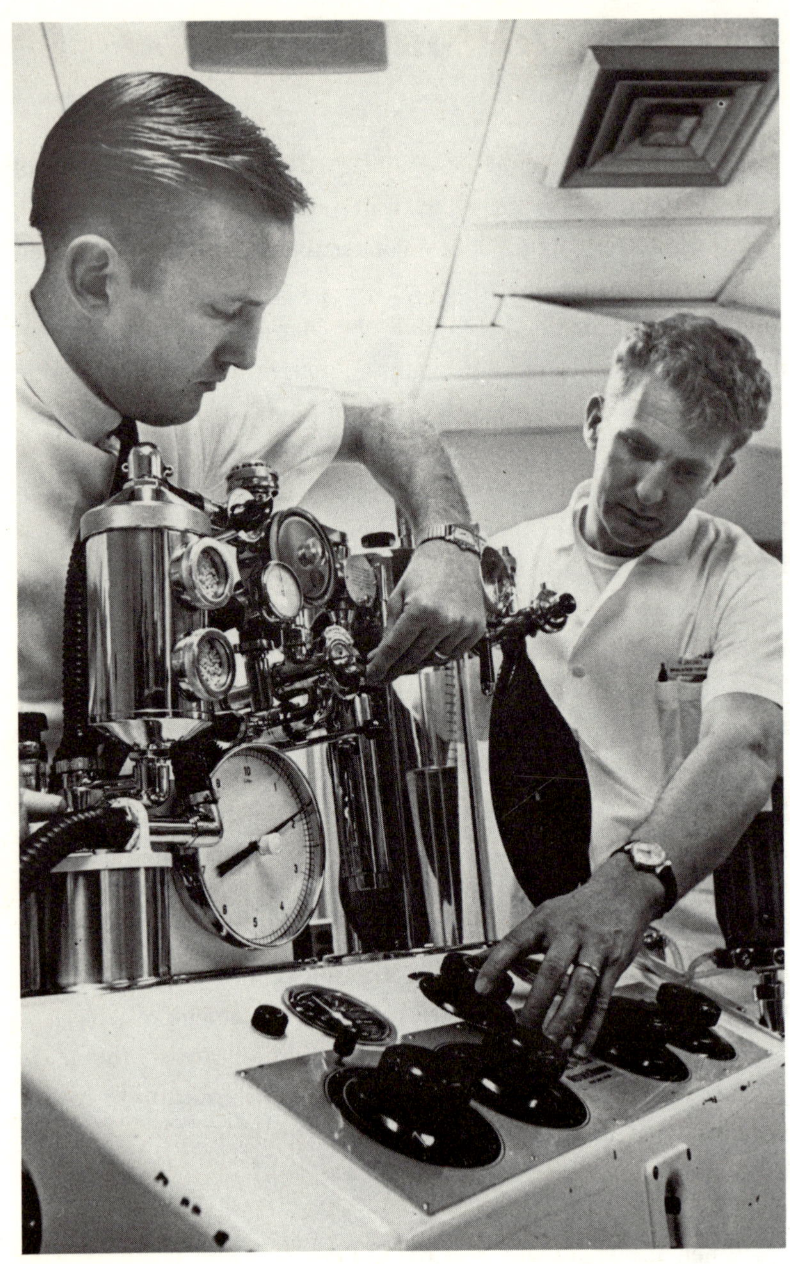

The inhalation therapist checks his equipment.

Pharmacist

Anthony Vicidomini carefully put the medication into the intravenous bottle's solution. He saw the solution change color with the addition of the medication. He checked it against the color chart, and seeing that it was satisfactory, replaced the bottle cap. He then put a package of tubing with a needle attached in a protective plastic bag, and with tape attached the bag to the bottle of liquid. Next he checked the order sheet on the table next to him and the label on the drug he had added, then the name of the patient whose order sheet he was working on. Satisfied that all was in order, he removed the bottle and bag from under the shield, placed a label on it that stated the patient's name, room number, and the drug and amount that was added to the solution. Anthony added his own name and date, placed the equipment in a large plastic bag, twisting the tie-wire around it. He then put the entire setup to one side of his work counter.

Anthony Vicidomini is a registered pharmacist who works in a hospital. Part of his daily routine is to make up intravenous solutions that will be administered to patients during the day. It is only a small part of his daily activities.

To become a pharmacist, a student must take a five-year college program. After graduation, Anthony had served a one-year apprenticeship in another hospital, and then had come to his present hospital to work as a licensed pharmacist in one of the satellite pharmacies established on the patient care units.

The concept of satellite pharmacy is relatively new. Anthony found that working within one was very much like being a chief pharmacist. His contact with the doctors was direct and he enjoyed his discussions with them and the nursing staff on the unit.

Another part of his work within the satellite pharmacy was

NATIONAL ASSOCIATION:

American Association for Inhalation Therapists
3554 9th Street
Riverside, California 92501

Nursing Aide and Orderly

Margaret Fleming wheeled the cart down the hall, delivering fresh ice water to each patient on her unit. She had worked in the hospital for three years and had transferred from the housekeeping department to the nursing department only four months ago. As part of her training in the nursing department she had taken classes in nursing aide routines and skills. It might seem that disbursing ice water to patients requires no particular skill or knowledge, but this is actually not true. Many patients in a hospital are on a routine called "intake and output." This means that their total consumption of food and fluid has to be noted on a special chart and accounted for completely. In addition, their output of urine has to be measured carefully to give the medical staff a record of how their bodies are maintaining a balance between their intake and output of fluid. Margaret kept the intake and output records on a number of the patients. Her job was time-consuming and very important.

Being a nursing aide is a serious and important job in a hospital. Many of the comfort and care measures given to patients are carried out by the nursing aide or her counterpart, the nursing male orderly.

The need for nursing aides and orderlies has been increasing steadily over the years. Most nursing aides and orderlies are paid while they receive on-the-job training in the hospital. The classes, lasting from three to six months, are given by professional nurses, often assisted by practical nurses.

Simple tasks such as transporting a patient by stretcher or wheel chair require an understanding of how to move or lift a patient, both for the safety and care of the patient and the safety and health of the aide. The students are taught proper body

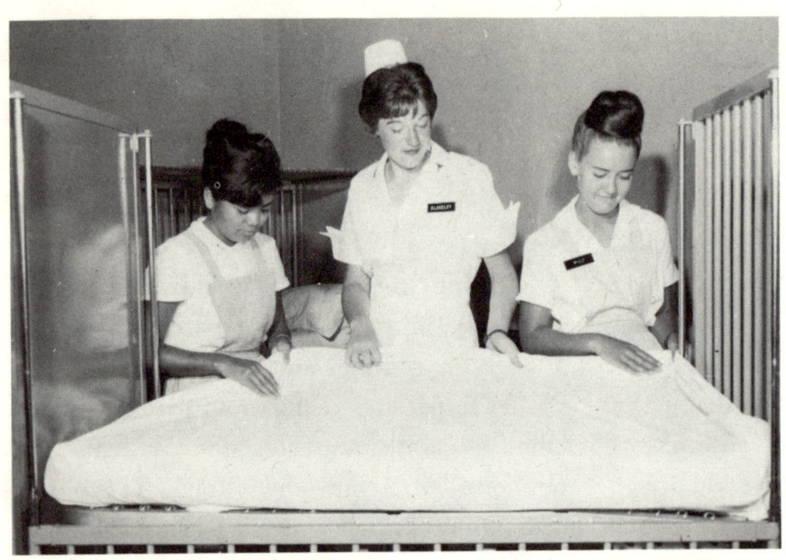

Training nursing aides

movements, the use of various items of equipment, and methods of working with each patient.

Classes for nursing aides offer the employee an opportunity for advancement. In many hospitals there are differences in both pay and duties for various classifications of the aides and orderlies.

REQUIREMENTS: high school education desirable but not necessary

COURSE OF STUDY: Basic nursing care, including bed-making, transportation of patients, temperature- and pulse-taking, bathing and feeding of patients, supply and equipment maintenance, safety measures, recording information on record forms

NATIONAL ASSOCIATION: There is no national association for nursing aides and orderlies. For more information contact your local hospital.

Dietician

One of the very first doctor's orders written on a patient's hospital chart concerns his diet in the hospital. If there are no medical problems relating to his food, he is placed on a "regular" diet. In hospital jargon that means that a patient can eat whatever he wishes to select from the hospital menu.

Providing food for the many hospitalized patients in any institution is no easy task. Not only are there a wide variety of specialized diets that must be prepared, but the tastes and preferences of a large number of people must be considered in the overall selection of food.

The person in charge of this problem is a trained dietician. No one is more familiar with a patient's complaints than this member of the health team. The chief dietician in a hospital is very much like someone with an extremely large family, none of whom likes the same thing, wants the same thing, or can eat the same thing at any given time!

Planning a hospital menu requires a great deal of skill. Not only must the dietician know the nutritional value of many foods, but must also plan menus based on the availability of any food at a given period. When planning is properly organized, the dietician uses vegetables currently in plentiful supply at a reasonable price. Meats, poultry, eggs, bread, fruits, and vegetables, as well as many other items, are purchased by a hospital in great quantities. A knowledgeable dietician is up-to-date on the wholesale price of every item to be purchased, and will plan menus with an eye on the market conditions of foods.

Planning meals economically is only a small part of the dietician's work. Meals must be balanced and nourishing as well. The dietician must have an organizational ability to work with the many people attached to the department. In a large hospital there may be a great number of dieticians and personnel working under the direction of a chief dietician.

To become a dietician, a young man or woman must take a college course specializing in foods and nutrition offered at many universities and colleges all over the country. On completion, the graduate dietician is required to complete a one-year internship in a hospital or a restaurant chain operation accredited with the American Dietetic Association.

There are many different areas of specialization in dietetics. A graduate may be interested in the administrative end. This means purchasing, management or personnel, and other administrative details. A graduate may prefer therapeutic activities, working directly with people. An example would be working with a group of schoolchildren who must be taught how to live with a particular disease, such as diabetes. A graduate dietician may prefer to teach dietetics to interns, nurses, and other health care team members. Dieticians also work on research units, developing new and different techniques to be used in conjunction with other medical therapies. Some may work in the out-patient clinic of a hospital or in a free-standing clinic, not directly associated with a hospital or medical center. They explain how best to use foods for nutritional standards and how to work that food into a tight budget.

REQUIREMENTS: high school education

COURSE OF STUDY: Major in nutrition and food courses, Institution Management, Chemistry, Bacteriology, Physiology, Mathematics, and Social Sciences

NATIONAL ASSOCIATION:

The American Dietetic Association
620 N. Michigan Avenue
Chicago, Illinois 60611

Operating Room Technician

The surgery schedule was completed at Billowbrook General Hospital. No one was more elated by the day's events than George Herman. Today had been his first time as scrub technician with the chief of surgery.

Ever since high school, George had wanted to become a doctor. However, his family was large and money was very difficult to come by. His high school advisor had suggested that George look into possible hospital training in a related area of health care work. Military service cut into George's initial plans, but he had been assigned to the medical corps and was given an education as a corpsman while in the army.

After completing military service, George checked with his community hospital and found it had an active program for training surgical assistants. He signed up at once and began his training under the Department of Surgery. Every day George would report on duty an hour before the regular surgical schedule began. He would "pick instruments" with the help of the professional operating room nurses who taught him each instrument's name and use. After picking the right instruments and in the right numbers for the particular operation that he was assigned to, George would "scrub up." He would don his sterile gown and gloves and place the sterilized instruments properly on his surgical table.

Working with the nurse that was assigned to teach him the various operative techniques, George would then assist the now ready physicians to don their gowns and gloves, and prepare the patient for operation. Standing beside the teaching nurse, George would observe what she handed to each doctor and when, how she held the instrument, what she did with it when the doctor had finished using it, and other important details.

Within a short period George was taking the teaching nurse's position, and she in turn watched him to be sure that he was doing everything correctly. Soon afterward, he was assigned to surgical procedures that he had shown he was capable of handling without a supervisory staff member. Within six months George was able to work at almost every surgical procedure carried out at the hospital. He was totally familiar with all the instrumentation used, the various suture materials, needles and blade sizes, and numerous other important details of surgical scrub work.

Today's scrub had been the "graduation" experience for him. He had scrubbed with the chief of surgery and had been complimented on his performance.

Surgical technicians had their start during World War II. After the war, many went back into civilian life and found opportunities for employment in hospitals all over the country. It was soon recognized that these technicians could fill a great need within the hospital. Previously, nurses were used to assist the physician in the operating room. As more and more areas of specialized techniques demanded the use of the professional nurses, they were replaced by trained surgical technicians.

Many of the technicians are men, but a great many are women, who have taken courses in surgical techniques. The majority of major hospitals and medical centers all over the country are now using the services of surgical technicians in their operating rooms.

Training courses vary in length in individual institutions, but are rarely less than six months. Men and women with military training in surgical techniques are usually given preference for admission.

On completion of the basic program the graduate technician will work on approximately five to nine operations per day, depending on the type of surgery. Complicated and delicate

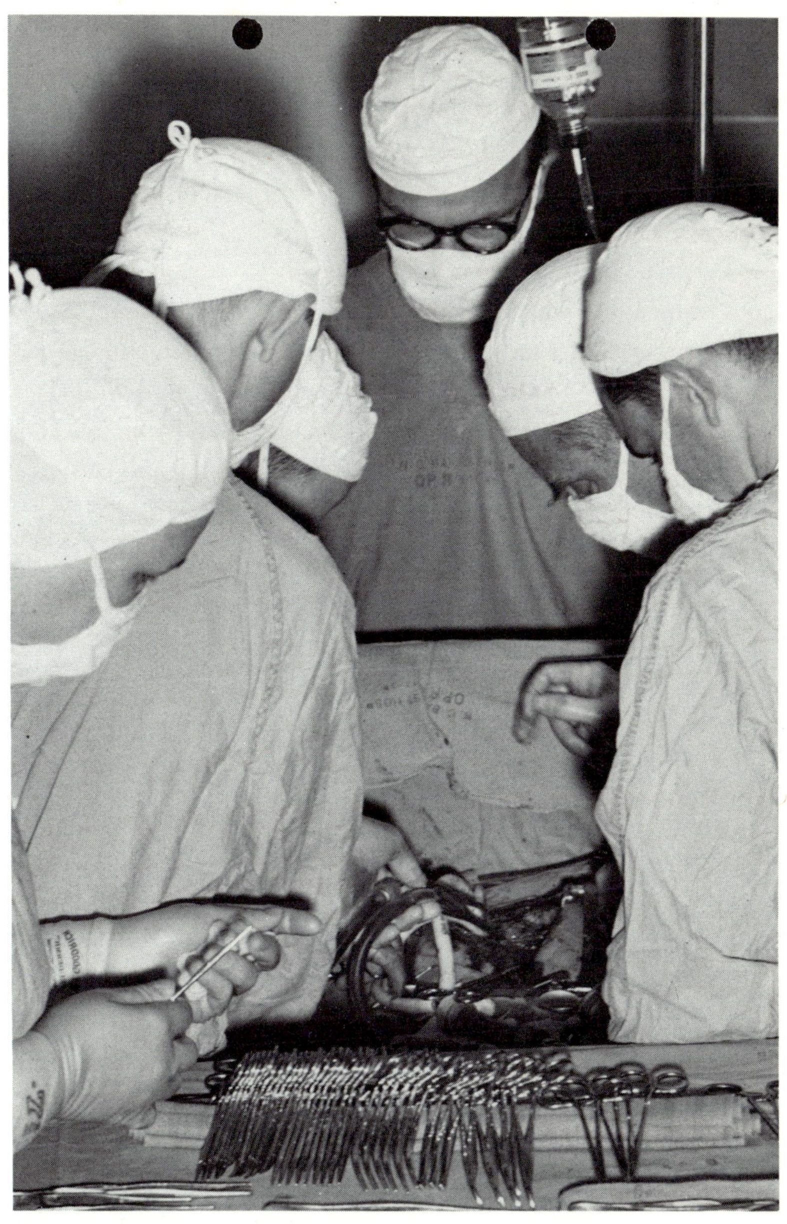

The operating-room technician must know the use of many instruments.

operations on the brain take a much greater amount of time, of course, than does the removal of an appendix.

Specialization in one particular type of surgery is also a possibility for a trained technician. He may request to be assigned to a specialization area and gain experience through exposure to procedures in that specialty.

REQUIREMENTS: high school education

COURSE OF STUDY: History of Surgery, English Communications, Terminology, Ethical, Legal, Moral Responsibilities, Anatomy and Physiology, Microbiology, Drugs and Solutions, Patient Care, Principles of Operating Room Technique, and Surgical Procedures (Montefiore Hospital and Medical Center, Bronx, New York)

NATIONAL ASSOCIATION:

Association of Operating Room Nurses
8085 E. Prentice Avenue
Englewood, Colorado 80110

preparing unit doses of medication for the patients assigned to his area. Some patients received medication every three or four hours, some only once a day. Some of the medications were injectable and others required the patient to take them by mouth, intravenously, or by another means depending on the particular condition and illness.

Working with the nurses on the units, Anthony found that the satellite pharmacy was a great help to them in obtaining updated information about drug therapy, new drugs currently in use, and their actions on the patients. And the nurses were a great help to him in discussions of particular patient problems relating to the medication administration methods. Weekly conferences were held by the pharmacists and the nursing staff of various units discussing drugs in use on the units and the shared responsibility of the doctor, nurse, and pharmacist relative to the patients they were treating.

In the main pharmacy located in another area of the hospital, the chief pharmacist and his assistants provided the various drugs and medicaments necessary to all parts of the hospital. It was their job to purchase, inventory, and disburse the materials to the satellite pharmacies, such as Anthony's.

In the clinic area of the hospital, another pharmacy and pharmacist provided services to the ambulatory patients that came to the clinic. Here prescriptions for drugs, salves, liquids, compounds, and other medicaments were processed daily. The pharmacist on duty was often called upon for consultation with the physician and the patient and nurse to work out the best solution to a problem. Young men and women entering the field of pharmacy will find a challenging frontier of health care.

REQUIREMENTS: high school education

COURSE OF STUDY: English, Mathematics, Chemistry, Physics, Zoology, Biology, Social Sciences, and professional courses dealing with chemical medicines, pharmaceutical chemistry, pharmacy practice, and laboratory instruction (University of North Carolina)

NATIONAL ASSOCIATION:

American Pharmaceutical Association
2215 Constitution Avenue N.W.
Washington, D.C. 20037

Physical Therapist

Nancy Dunning carefully supported the patient's right leg as he pushed his left leg hard against the bedboard. After repeating the exercise ten times, Nancy let the patient rest a few moments, and then supported his left leg while he did the exercise with his right one.

This particular patient had had a cerebral vascular accident, commonly called a "stroke." During his initial, critical period of illness, he had been paralyzed in his legs, and had developed a slight speech impediment. Several weeks later, most of the movement and control of his legs had returned. The speech impediment still remained, however, and he was working with a speech therapist. Nancy's job was to help the patient gain back the strength and control over his limbs that had diminished during the long weeks of inactivity and paralysis. The exercise program she had planned included sessions such as she had just completed, as well as walking between parallel bars and some light weightlifting. Each day the patient practiced with the therapist and often by himself in his room.

Cerebral accident patients are only one of the many kinds of people cared for by a physical therapist. Many patients who require physical therapy have had severe injuries resulting from falls or car accidents. In situations where a limb has been amputated, the patient has to be taught to function with an artificial device. In other illnesses, such as arthritis, spinal cord injuries, and similar conditions that cause a dysfunction or total impairment of a part of the body, the therapist will work with the patient to teach him how to adjust to his limitations and how to keep his body in good physical condition, regardless of the impairment.

The therapist has an important role in his or her contact

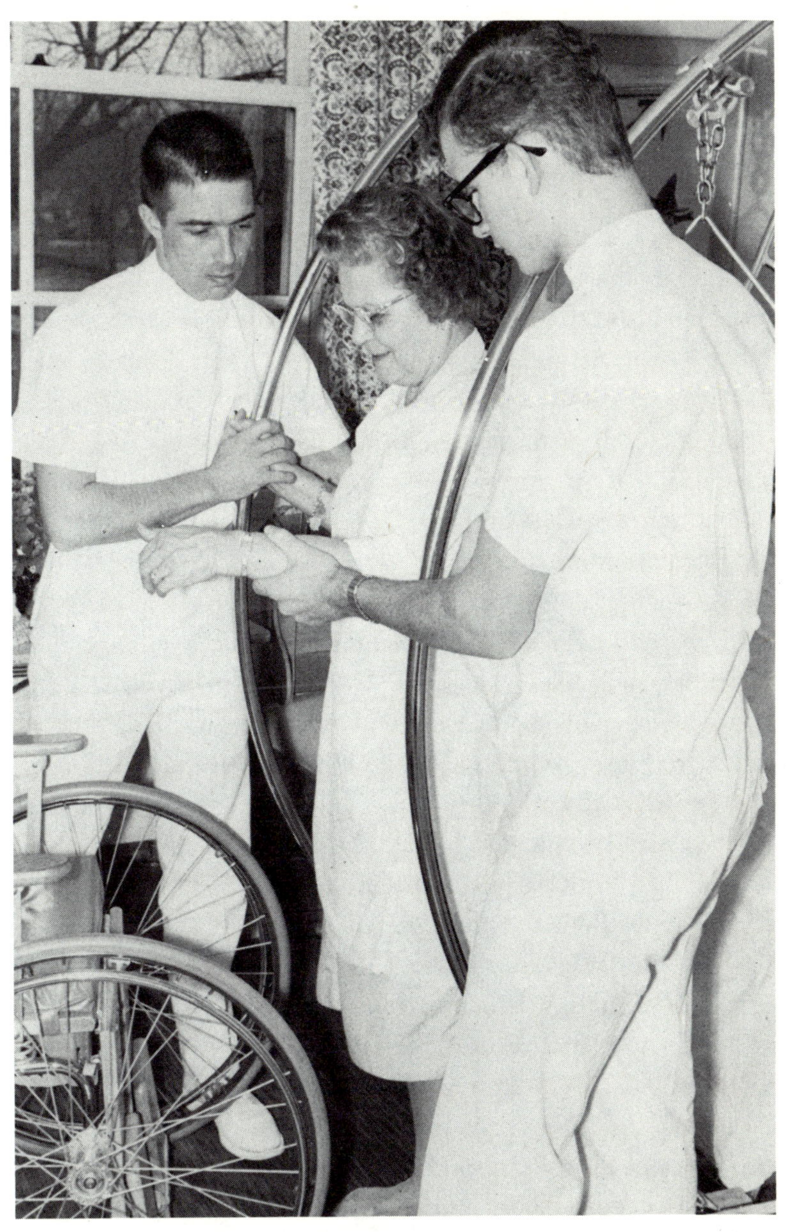

The physical therapist often works with patients who have suffered injuries from falls or car accidents.

with the patient. Often, it is the therapist that the patient responds to initially, even more than to the doctors or nurses, since the therapist represents the "outside world" where the patient will eventually have to live and function. If the therapist were to show horror or dismay at the patient's affliction, the patient would feel that this is the way the world would view him, too.

One of the most challenging aspects of the physical therapist's job is the opportunity to develop new ways to help patients. What is just the right splint or crutch to use, or should something new be designed for a particular need? In Nancy's case, working closely with physicians and nurses, she had redesigned a hand crutch for a woman whose arm was impaired as the result of a stroke. The crutch, fitted to the disabled hand of the patient, gave total support to the fingers and wrist, yet allowed the hand to assume normal positions when properly placed on hard or soft surfaces. The attachments to the arm were made of leather and looked like a wide wristband. The finger attachments were scooped-out ovals that allowed each finger to rest within the cup. From the back the limb looked normal. The patient herself had worked with Nancy in developing the materials for the crutch. She had suggested the use of plastic glove dryers as their first working model. Nancy had obtained them through a local store. Both she and the patient worked at the design of the crutch in their daily sessions.

Nancy Dunning is one of thousands of physical therapists working with handicapped patients in hospitals, clinics, and rehabilitation centers throughout the country. Their work is vital in the long-range recovery of many patients with major disabilities. Without the therapists' help these patients would often not be able to keep up their normal activities as well as they do.

To become a physical therapist, a student must take a four-year college course, and then must pass an exam to become licensed.

REQUIREMENTS: high school education

COURSE OF STUDY: Physics, General Chemistry, Biologic Sciences, Psychology, Speech, Human Gross Anatomy, Human Physiology, Pathology, Therapeutic Exercise, History, Administration, Economics and Ethics of Health Care, Psychology of Work and Disability, Clinical Education (University of Texas Medical School at Dallas)

NATIONAL ASSOCIATION:

American Physical Therapists Association
1156 15th Street NW
Washington, D.C. 20005

Speech Therapist

Another vital team member in the care of patients is the speech therapist, or pathologist. Unknown to the majority of patients in a hospital, the speech therapist works with a small group of patients who require highly specialized skills in speech techniques. The patients include children and adults. Their illnesses range from brain damage at birth to injury to the speech centers due to a stroke.

John Stephen had suffered a severe stroke many months ago. He had only partially recovered. His major concern was not his inability to walk, but his inability to communicate clearly. His words came out garbled and slurred, and he was often frustrated to the point of rage because he could not make himself understood.

Ann Cherny, speech therapist, had begun working with John Stephen before he left the hospital. Slowly, she made him aware of the help that she could offer. Soon he looked forward to his sessions with her and worked hard at practicing the sounds and exercises she gave to him.

Speech therapists or pathologists earn a master's degree in colleges and universities. The courses are aimed at preparing the student to work with various types of speech impairments.

Many speech pathologists are also trained in audiology, the science of hearing. Hearing impairments in young children are often discovered through tests administered in the public school systems. Many are referred to audiologists, who work with the child in lip-reading methods and other devices.

REQUIREMENTS: high school education

COURSE OF STUDY: English, Sociology, Psychology, Mathematics, Political Science, Speech Pathology courses, Zoology, Statistics, Guidance and Counseling (University of Wyoming)

NATIONAL ASSOCIATION:

American Speech and Hearing Association
9030 Old Georgetown Road
Washington, D.C. 20014

Physician's Associate

One of the newest careers in health care is demanding, challenging, and rapidly growing in importance. This is the role of the physician's associate. Programs to train this health care team member have sprung up at medical centers throughout the country, and young men and women are fast becoming interested.

Dick Sheltz is a graduate physician's associate. He and his family moved to Nome, Alaska, two years after he completed his course at Duke University in Durham, North Carolina. Dick had chosen Alaska because he believed it would give him the fullest opportunity to use his training. He is responsible for the health care services given to people in a one-hundred-mile radius of his home base. Traveling by plane or jeep, he is the only medically trained person in his entire area. He keeps in communication with his base clinic by radio.

The doctors who employ Dick set up the base clinic and hired four physician's associates to work with them. The duties of the physician's associates include preventive as well as emergency health care. They deliver babies, set broken bones, diagnose physical ailments, and prescribe medications and treatments. Their communication system with the physicians provides back-up information and help.

The first program for physician's associates was started at Duke University in 1965. Since that time many other medical centers have begun similar programs. Requirements for admission differ, but all applicants must be high school graduates. Preference is given in most situations to students with two years of college credits, military medical corps training, or a related medical field background such as medical technology or nursing.

Developing skills in very technical procedures and diag-

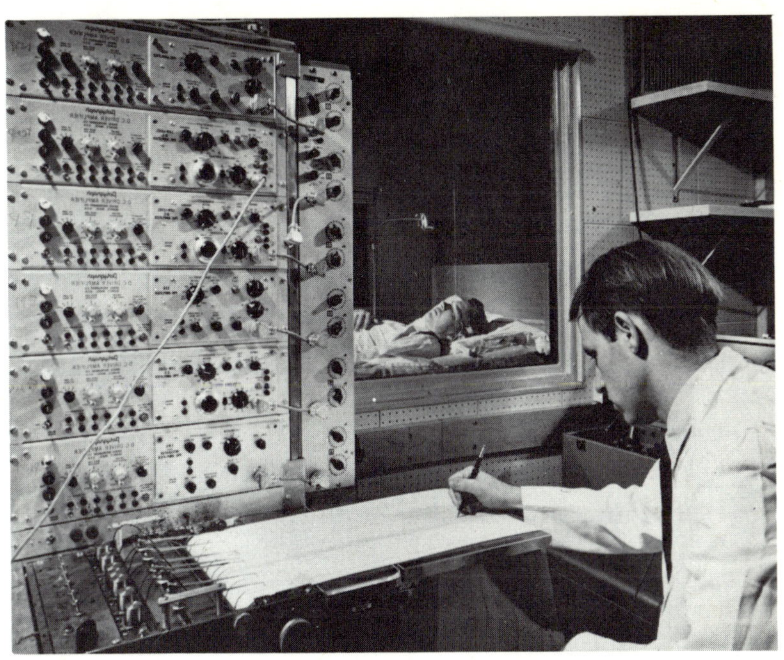

The physician's associate at work

nostic testing methods, the students work under the direct supervision of a physician or a group of physicians to whom they are responsible. Classes are taught by graduate physician's associates and professional nurses and physicians. In many of the programs the students are assigned to special projects. Working in a clinic with specific responsibilities for patient care, such as taking medical histories and doing physical examinations, carrying out blood tests, or assisting in technical diagnostic procedures, the student physician's associate learns how to work on various levels within the health care field, as well as how to relate to the individual patient and his family.

The programs vary not only in content, but in length. (The course at Duke University, for instance, is two years long.) Some prepare the assistant to act only as an aide to the doctor, while others promote depth in knowledge and skills so that the graduate often assumes many of the previous responsibilities of the physician, under his supervision.

REQUIREMENTS: high school education, previous experience or training in the health field

COURSE OF STUDY: Analysis of Health Systems Development, Anatomy and Physiology, Chemical Biology and Pharmacology, Clinical Diagnosis, Objective Medicine, Clinical Medicine, Patient Evaluation, Human Growth and Development, plus a clinical curriculum of 36 weeks of required clinical rotations and 24 weeks of elective clinical rotations (Duke University, Durham, North Carolina)

NATIONAL ASSOCIATION:

Association of Physician's Associates
Box 2914 CHS
Duke University Medical Center
Durham, North Carolina 27706

Hospital Administrator

Hospital administration is a relatively new career in the health care field. Up until the early 1960's, most hospitals or other health care institutions were administered by physicians. The complexity of modern hospitals soon required a special training. While many hospitals are still supervised overall by medical directors, the hospital administrator, who is trained in business rather than medicine, has become a vital link in the chain of responsibility.

Hospital administration is often divided into special areas of responsibility and authority. Since there are so many vital components to a hospital, it would almost be impossible for any one person to be responsible for all the inner workings and problems. In a large medical center there may be an administrator in charge of the clinics, another in charge of the operating room department, and still others in charge of various medical/nursing divisions, such as Surgery, Medicine, Pediatrics, and Obstetrics. Administrative personnel may be found in such areas as Planning Divisions, Public Relations and Fund Raising, or Research and Development.

Health care administration today is a diverse and interesting field. Clinics, the new future in health care, have specific problems within themselves that are very often different from the hospital. This new field is opening to administrative-minded people who wish to work in a health care career.

Owen Fife is a hospital administrator. He received a master's degree from Columbia University in New York City after completing his undergraduate program at the University of Kentucky. A typical example of the hospital administrator's work is the problem that Owen faced when he reported for work one day. It involved the chief of one of his medical services. The hospital was building a new wing for a particular specialty. Doctors who specialized in these particular patients would be all in one area, with equipment and personnel especially geared for the patients. Owen agreed with this arrangement. However, he also knew that if the beds were not kept full with specialty patients, he could not allow them to remain empty if other patients needed admission. The doctor in charge wanted the beds *strictly* for his specialty; Owen wanted them *primarily* for the specialty, but not limited if there were too few patients on the unit to fill them.

Owen was finally able to solve the problem through a suggestion offered by the director of nursing. She proposed that he take one of the already functioning units of the hospital and make it into a test specialty unit. If what Owen thought was true — that the specialty would not fill the unit — this fact could be shown to the doctor who would be in charge of the new wing.

The problems of administering a hospital are numerous and often not as easily solved as the one just described. The many specialty units in the hospital are fiercely competitive; the staff of physicians is constantly seeking new and different ways of treating patients; the community often demands of the hospital more than it is able to provide; the patients and their families understandably are equally demanding; and the problem of running in the black gets harder every day.

A hospital administrator is sort of a combined business manager and referee. He must tie together the many areas in the hospital so that they function together and yet separately in their own right. He must be open to new ideas. He must also be sensitive to the problems of the community. He attends community meetings, works with city or country health officials and often with many other city agencies.

The administrator of a hospital clinic may become more involved in community problems than does the hospital itself.

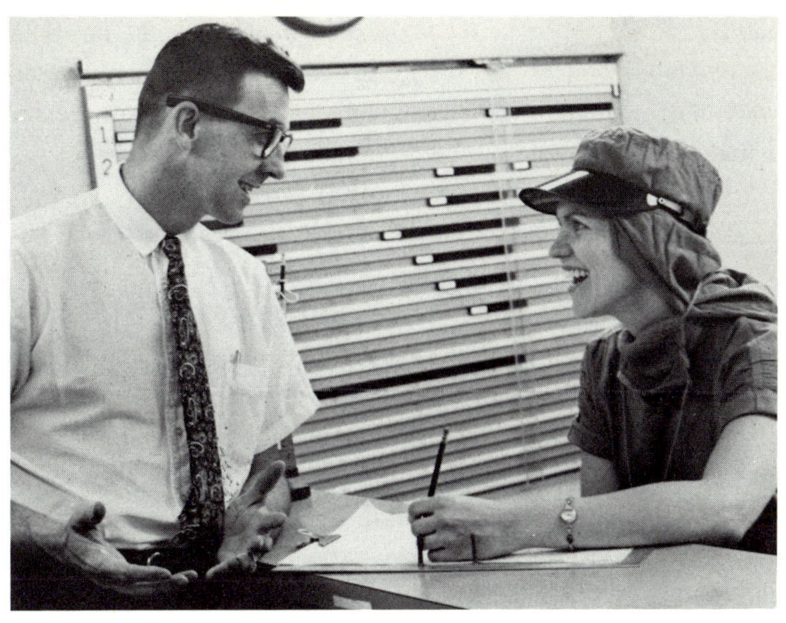

The hospital administrator is a sort of combined business manager and referee.

The clinic manager is often in administrative charge of the emergency room, which provides medical assistance on an emergency basis. Frequently, its successful operation will make the difference between good or bad relations with the community.

The problems of the various specialty units within the hospital often ultimately come to the administrator. Perhaps there is an idea for purchasing new types of beds, chairs, or instruments, or redesigning the unit itself. Working closely with the nursing and medical staffs of the specialty unit, the administrator establishes policies and procedures that are important to the unit's operation.

In public health administration the administrator of a community clinic will be actively engaged in meeting the needs of the community in preventive health care, teaching methods related to drug abuse, infant care, home care for the aged, dietary management, and many other community related projects.

The hospital administrator's job requires a master's degree. Most programs demand an internship of at least one year. During this time the student works in a hospital, nursing home, or clinic in a related role of administrative intern. Many hospitals provide rotational periods of experience for the intern so that he will gain information and knowledge of various areas of responsibility. In public health administration, the internship may be taken at any of the many government-sponsored clinical services, including those on Indian reservations and in Federal prisons.

REQUIREMENTS: high school education plus college degree graduate program

COURSE OF STUDY: Health Care Facilities Organization and Management, Social and Economic Aspects of Health Care, Administration of Extended Care Facilities, Mental Health Care Administration, Organizational Behavior and Health Care Administration, Health Care Planning, Urban Health Services Research, Field Experience for Urban Health Trainees, Financial Management for Health Care Administration (University of Texas, San Antonio)

NATIONAL ASSOCIATION:

Association of University Programs in Hospital Administration
Suite 420
1 Dupont Circle
Washington, D.C. 20036

Hospital Maintenance Worker

The plans for the new hospital wing lay on the counter. The administrator had called for a meeting of all maintenance department members. He presented the plans for the new wing, explained why it had been designed as it had been, and what the building schedule would be. Then he opened the meeting for questions.

Rusty Damerson asked if the power generator currently providing emergency power for the hospital could absorb the new building's lighting system in an emergency. The administrator replied that an additional generator was to be incorporated into the new wing to handle that problem. Someone else said that from the drawing it looked like the closets for the mops and pails needed to keep the new wing clean were very small. The administrator jotted down a notation. Another man suggested that the lighting fixtures be kept a certain size throughout to permit easier purchasing and storage of fixture replacements and bulbs. The administrator made another notation.

Hospital maintenance workers such as Rusty Damerson carry out the often overlooked job of making sure that things are kept in proper working order. It is not an easy task. Hospitals function twenty-four hours a day, seven days a week throughout the year. There are very few rooms in a hospital that are not in constant use. Fixing a pipe, repairing a light, patching a wall, or painting it all must be done in a hurry.

Many hospital maintenance people take special training courses to work with some of the highly technical equipment used in the hospital. Most of the men in Rusty's department had graduated from commercial high schools. Many are trained

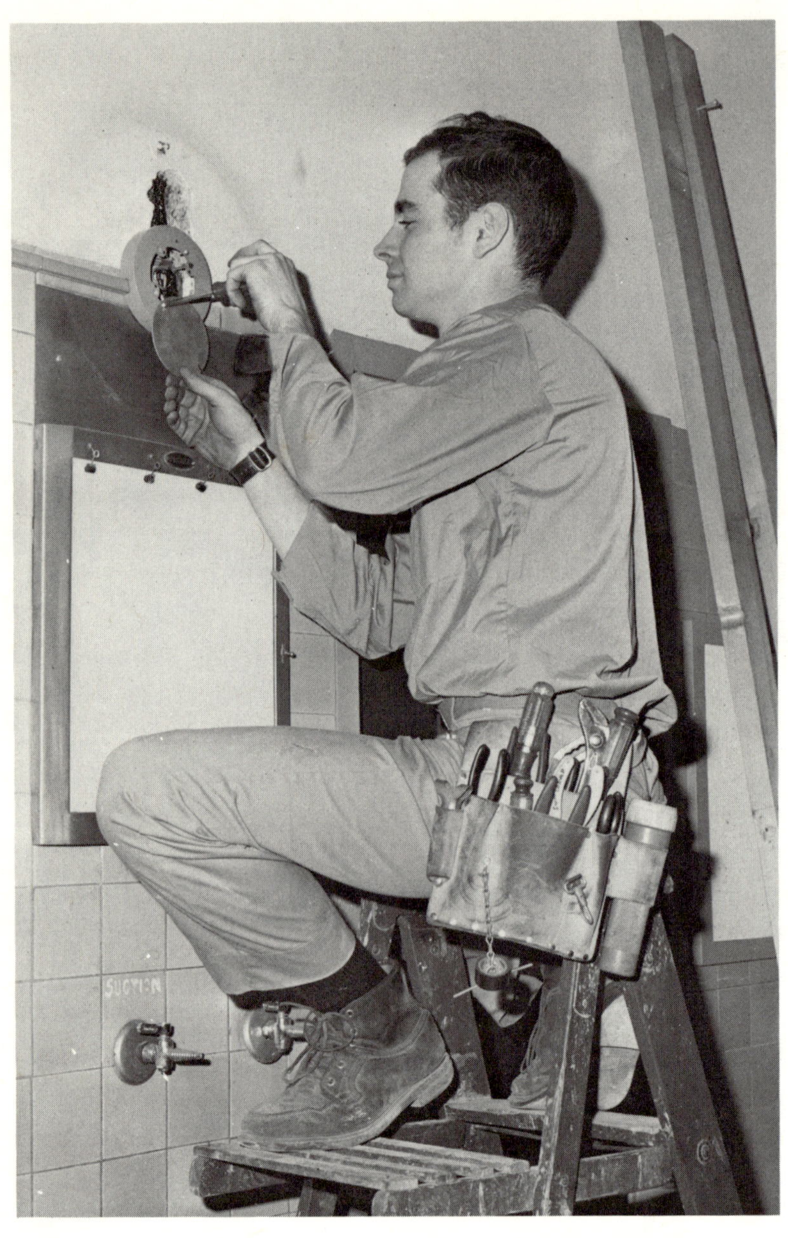

Hospital maintenance workers keep the hospital functioning twenty-four hours a day.

electricians, plumbers, or carpenters. A trained and experienced maintenance crew makes a big difference to the efficiency of the hospital. This career opens many opportunities to a young worker.

REQUIREMENTS: some kind of maintenance experience or vocational training

There is no national association for hospital maintenance workers. Contact your local hospital for more information in this area.

Housekeeper in the Hospital

Dan Hurter is chief housekeeper in a large hospital. His department employs over 150 people to see that the hospital is kept clean at all hours of the day and night, that there are adequate linens for all departments, including the operating rooms and clinics, as well as supplies for the staff and patients. In one month this hospital uses about 14 cases of soap (each case contains 3,000 bars); 51 cases of paper towels (5,000 towels to a case); 50 gallons of floor wash mix; 20 gallons of special floor wax; and 863 one-hundred-watt bulbs; and those are just a few of the items that Dan's department stocks, uses, and supplies.

Hospital housekeeper is not very often thought of as a possible career by a young man or woman. Yet the field is challenging and calls for interested people. A high school education is necessary, and courses in hotel or motel management are often very beneficial.

New methods of building construction, as well as new materials, have made the housekeeper's job a constantly changing one. The use of disposable linens, plus the pre-packing of many materials such as syringes, needles, and instruments, have brought about a new approach to garbage disposal and methods of collection. Some hospitals have developed their own internal delivery system of all supplies and equipment via monorail through the whole institution.

The hospital's housekeeping staff must become familiar with many types of equipment, such as the hyberbaric tank, a sort of land-based submarine where high-pressure oxygen treatments are carried out. Working in clinics, nursing homes, mobile units, retirement homes, and special premature nurseries, as well as hospitals, the housekeeping staff, along with the chief

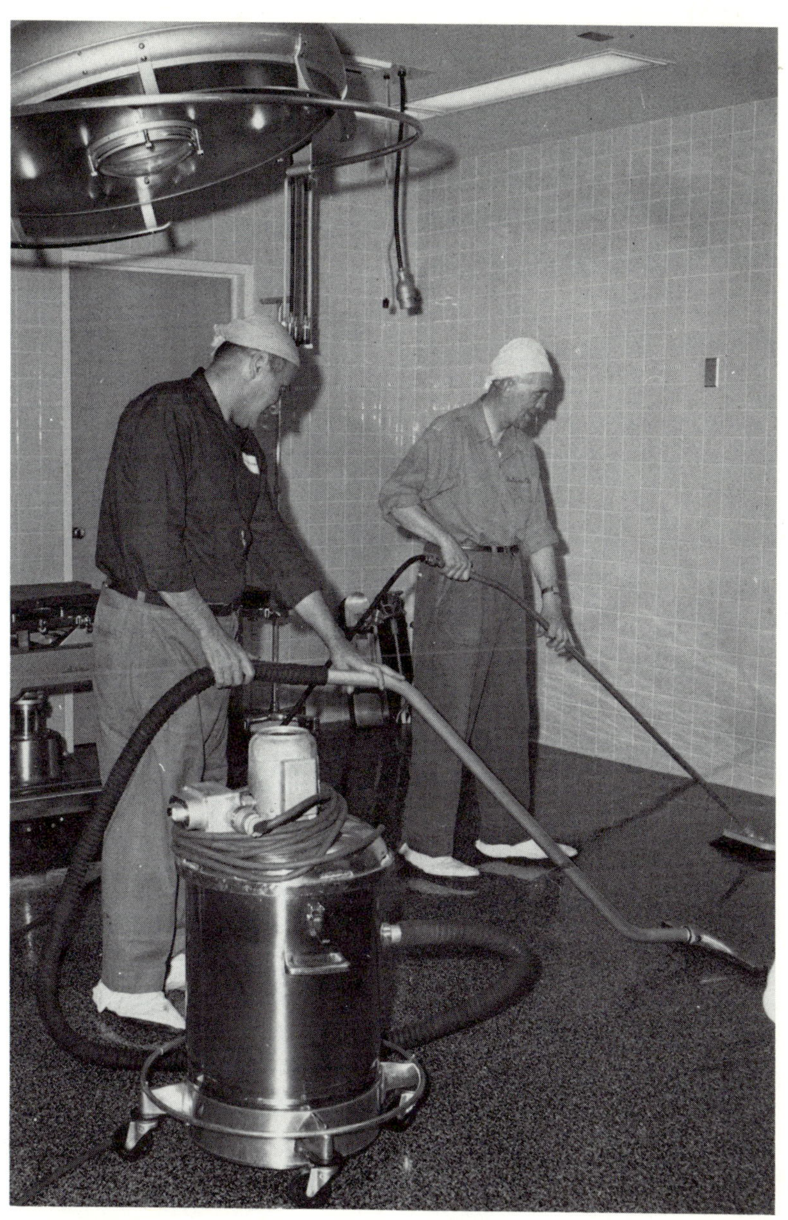

Keeping the operating room clean

housekeeper, must make sure that these units are clean at all times.

REQUIREMENTS: high school education, vocational programs in hotel or motel management

There is no national association for hospital housekeepers.

Record Librarian

Marjorie Peem, record librarian for a large city hospital, held a meeting with the newest members of her department. Over the years the medical record department had expanded until it now filled an entire floor of one wing of the hospital and used the services of some 15 staff personnel. The new staff members had all had some previous experience in medical record work.

The record room of any hospital is in many ways a nerve center of information. The records of patients previously admitted to the hospital or transferred from other hospitals are kept in this department. Some of the records are very lengthy and are microfilmed for storing. Microfilming has helped considerably with the vast storage problems that all hospitals contend with. In some states the law requires that a patient's chart be kept for at least seven years. Considering the fact that thousands and thousands of patients are admitted to hospitals throughout the United States in any year, the storage of just these records is a considerable problem. Microfilming allows the hospital to retain many more records than would be possible if the charts were kept in their usual 8½″ x 11″ folders.

The medical record librarian in a hospital can often make a great difference in effective care for a patient. Locating old records in a matter of moments when the patient is unconscious in the emergency room and unable to give any medical history will quickly aid the doctor in understanding the patient's condition. Filing charts and storing records are important parts of the job of the record librarian, but they are not all of the job by any means. Various agencies require vast amounts of statistics from all health care institutions. The record room must keep track of the number of patients admitted, their age, sex, religion, financial background, how long they stayed in the hospital, what surgery was performed, what drugs or blood transfusions were given, and other information as well.

Many universities and colleges offer courses in library science. The program requires two years of graduate study. During the two years of graduate study the student specializes in the medical field.

REQUIREMENTS: high school education

COURSE OF STUDY: Medical Terminology, Medical Record Science, Hospital Organization, Departmental Organization and Management, Medicolegal Aspects of Records, lectures on fundamentals of medical science, anatomy, and physiology (graduate study, University Medical Center, Jackson, Mississippi)

NATIONAL ASSOCIATION:

Committee on Education and Registration
American Medical Record Association
Suite 1850
875 N. Michigan Avenue
Chicago, Illinois 60611

Social Worker

Eve Clayton used the few moments before the office opened to review her patient files for the day. Working at the psychiatric hospital social service department had been a new experience for her over the past year. She had previously worked for a community clinic, dealing with many types of problems — drug abuse, alcoholism, poverty, and many physical illnesses. Then one of the doctors had asked her to join the psychiatric hospital staff.

Eve wanted to become a clinical social worker in the field of mental health detection. Working in the community clinic, she had felt that she could make a contribution to helping people understand and adjust more readily to their everyday problems.

At the psychiatric hospital she was learning first hand of the impact that hospitalization of a family member in a mental institution had upon the entire family. She learned the various techniques of treatment, the supportive role that the staff and the patient's family must fulfill if the patient was to get better, and how much help was really needed.

There are many opportunities for social workers in this field. Government agencies rely heavily on social workers' reports for designating welfare, health, and housing and education programs. Many social workers prefer to work in the federal or local government programs because they feel that their efforts will make a significant contribution there. Others, working in hospitals, nursing homes, community agencies with drug and alcoholic programs, feel that they can help best by working directly with people in the community.

The majority of social workers are involved with the problems of the poor and underprivileged, but many aid other citizens as well. Social workers often work with the family of the

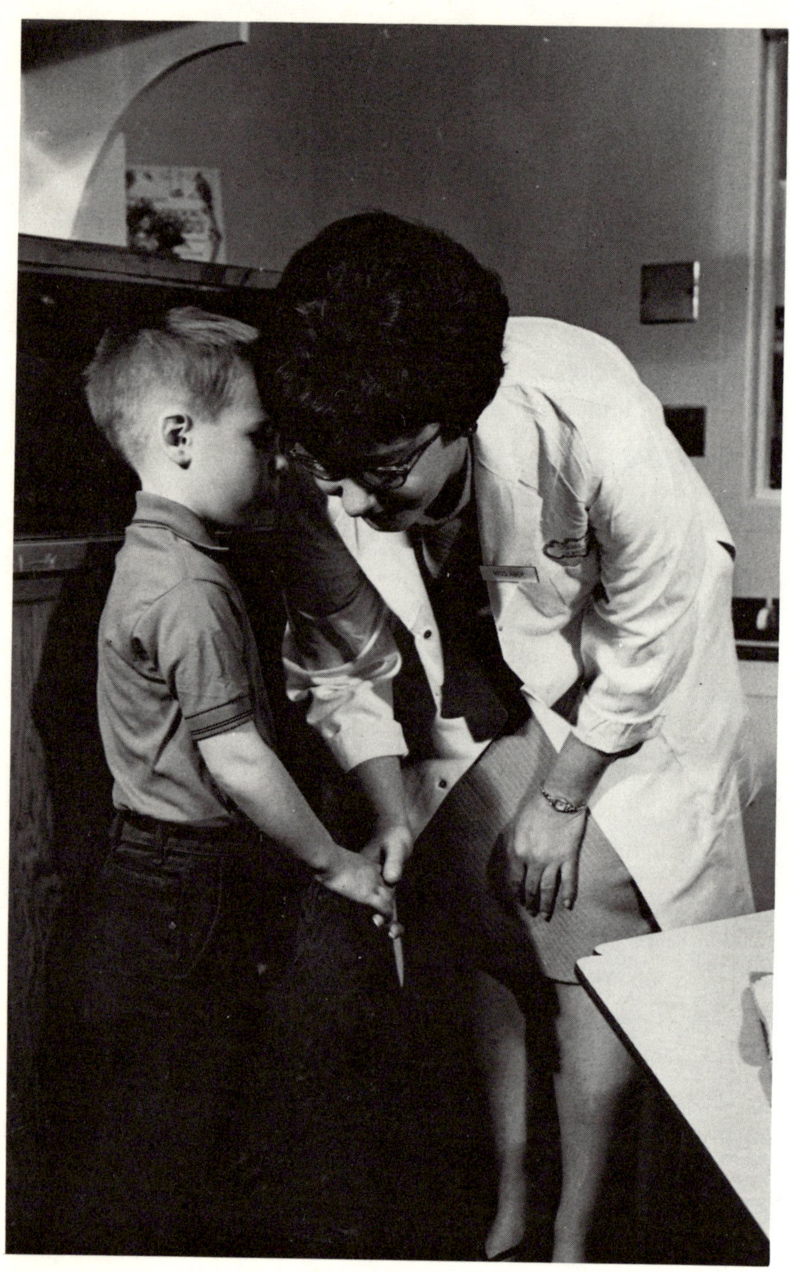

A social worker and a young patient

patient, as well as with the patient himself. Through the social worker's efforts, arrangements are made for home care assistance when a mother becomes hospitalized and her husband is unable to stay home and care for small children. Social workers often find housing for relatives of very sick people who are taken to distant hospitals for specialized care and treatment. They may provide meals, transportation, and other benefits for family members.

The social worker may work with the police and the family of a youthful offender of the law, providing counseling and guidance. Social workers help the physically handicapped to find jobs, housing, and assistance, to help them gain a productive place in society.

As a social worker, Eve Clayton prepared for her career in college. Mental health social work, community social work, hospital social work, and other areas are taught at the master's level in a college or university.

REQUIREMENTS: high school education

COURSE OF STUDY: Disorders of Development and Learning in Childhood, Perspectives on Human Behavior and Social Environment, Social Work Research Methods, Human Values and Social Problems, Social Work Services to Families, Psychopathology of Human Behavior, Small Group Theory, Marriage Counseling, Mental Retardation and Social Work, Social Work and the Law, Analysis of Social Service Systems (graduate study, School of Social Work, University of North Carolina)

NATIONAL ASSOCIATION:

Council on Social Work Education
345 E. 46th St.
New York, New York 10017

Dental Health Careers

Students interested in careers in dental health care have a wide variety of areas to choose from.

The profession of *dentistry* is taught at the college level. Admission requirements differ, but all schools require a good high school record. After completing the first three years of basic college courses, the student enrolls in dental school, a four-year program.

A *dental hygienist* performs such services as cleaning teeth, preparing diagnostic tests for the dentist, and counseling patients in oral health. Most hygienists work in private dental offices. The course leading to a certificate as a dental hygienist is two years long. There is also a four-year course leading to a college degree in dental hygiene.

A *dental laboratory technician* works in the dentist's office laboratory, a commercial dental laboratory, and sometimes in his own dental laboratory. He is a skilled mechanical technician, involved in making dentures. The training program is generally two years long.

A *dental assistant*, after a ten-to-twelve-month course, aids the dentist and assumes many responsibilities in the dentist's office. This is a fast-growing area for interested students. In some states the course may be two years long; in others students receive on-the-job training.

REQUIREMENTS: high school education for all four careers

COURSE OF STUDY

Dentistry: Biochemistry, Dental Ecology, Oral Biology, Oral Medicine, Microbiology, Restorative Dentistry, Surgery, Dental Ecology, Pharmacology, Orthodontics, Endodontics, Pedodontics, Preventive Dentistry, Anesthesia, Practice Administration (Dental School, University of North Carolina)

Dental Hygienist: Anatomy, Biochemistry, English, Dental-Anatomy Physiology, Dental Hygiene, Dental Materials and Techniques, Sociology, Speech, Dental Pharmacology, Clinical Dental Hygiene, Pathogenic Microbiology (Certificate Program, University of North Carolina)

Dental Laboratory Technician: Dental Anatomy and Physiology, Grammar, Dental Materials, Denture Techniques, Business Mathematics, Composition, Dental Metallurgy, Chemistry, Crown and Bridge Techniques, Physics, Ceramic Techniques, Dental Laboratory Practices, Jurisprudence and Ethics (Durham Technical Institute, Durham, North Carolina)

Dental Assistant: Dental Orientation, Secretarial Procedures, Preclinical Science Courses, Dental Materials, Clinical Services, Dental Techniques, Clinical Experience (University of North Carolina)

NATIONAL ASSOCIATION:

American Dental Association
211 E. Chicago Avenue
Chicago, Illinois 60611

Opticianry

Opticianry is the art of designing and fitting lenses and other devices for vision. The science of optics is a branch of physics and is concerned with study of light, the role of light in vision, and the geometry of light refraction and reflection.

The program for learning this skill is two years. Courses in mathematics, especially algebra and trigonometry, and physical sciences are important.

Ophthalmology is a specialty of medicine, and the preparation for becoming an ophthalmologist is similar to that of any doctor — premedical training, medical school, and residency programs in the specialty of ophthalmology.

REQUIREMENTS: high school education

COURSE OF STUDY: Technical Education, Grammar, Technical Math, Mechanical Optics, Properties of Matter, Lens Design and Sketching, Economics, English Composition, Geometric Optics, Oral Communications, Applied Psychology, Equipment Repair and Maintenance, Anatomy of the Eye, Physiology of the Eye, Contact Lenses (Opticianry, Durham Technical Institute, Durham, North Carolina)

NATIONAL ASSOCIATION:

American Association of Ophthalmology
1100 17th Street, NW
Washington, D.C. 20036

Business Worker in the Health Field

Although they are not often thought of in that way, hospitals, nursing homes, and other health care facilities are functioning businesses. Clerks, cashiers, accountants, comptrollers, insurance clerks, secretaries, receptionists, and others usually associated with the business field are employed in any health care institution.

Health care accounting is an interesting field for the young business-minded man or woman. Clerical work involves dealing with patients for admission, making payment arrangements, working with various insurance firms, health care programs, and government agencies.

A high school education, with emphasis on business skills, is usually required for work of this type in any health care institution.

Business workers are an important part of the hospital staff.

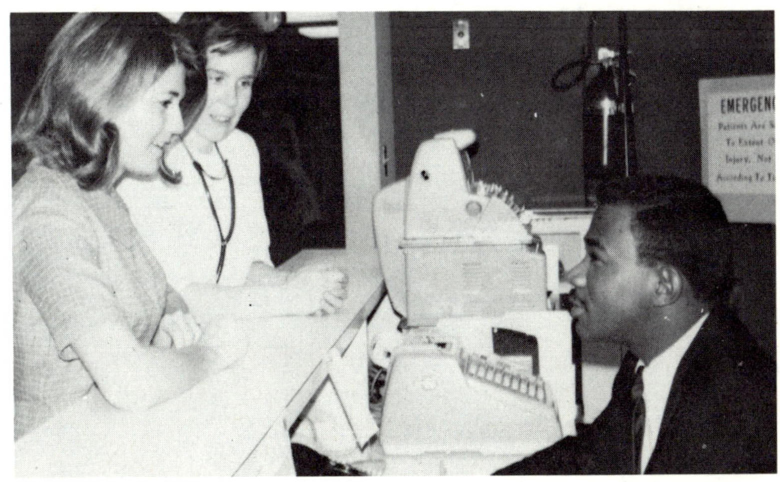

Health Care Planner

A young man or woman interested in studying architecture might well consider a career as a health care architect. Unfortunately, too few do. The many millions of dollars spent in new construction each year could be more fruitful if the planners and builders of health care facilities had greater understanding of the specific needs of these institutions.

Poor planning and even poor construction of facilities in the past has often made the costs of running these institutions higher than necessary.

Physicians, long the most important source of information relative to health care facility planning, sometimes have a one-sided view of the actual space needs and functions of the institution. Administrators, although highly trained, rarely have worked in all the areas of day-to-day operation for any length of time to understand the total picture.

Health care planners must be trained as architects. More and more planners are needed, and the field offers great opportunities for the interested student.

REQUIREMENTS: high school education

NATIONAL ASSOCIATION:

American Institute of Architects
1785 Massachusetts Avenue NW
Washington, D.C. 20036

Index

ABOUT THE AUTHOR

Eleanor Kay is a registered nurse who lives in Tuckahoe, New York. She received her nursing training at Flower Fifth Avenue Hospital in New York City. She has been associated with Gracie Square Hospital in New York City and Duke University Medical Center in Durham, North Carolina. The author has written a number of books for Franklin Watts, including *The First Book of Nurses, Nurses and What They Do, Let's Find Out About Hospitals,* and *Read About the School Nurse.*